Good Housekeeping

make the most of your lips

Jo Glanville-Blackburn

series editor
Vicci Bentley

HarperCollins*Illustrated*

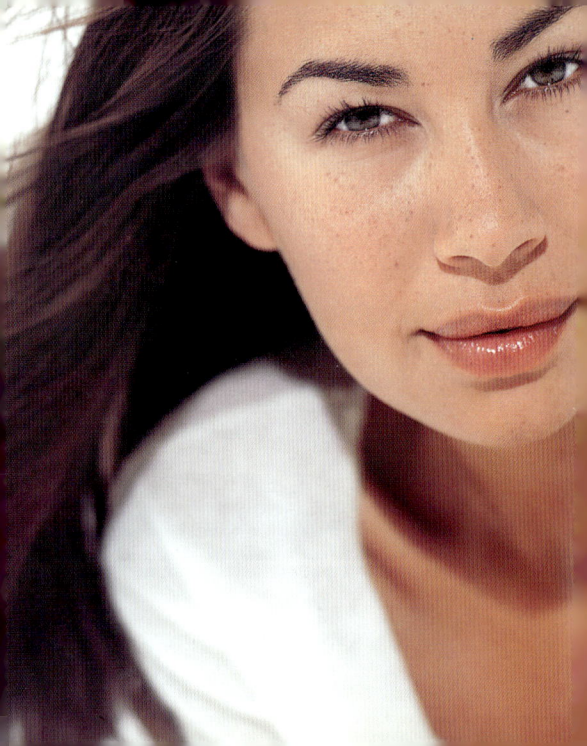

contents

introducing lips 6

looking after lips 14

lip work-outs 38

making-up lips 50

lip looks 82

'laughter is the shortest distance between two people.'

Victor Borge

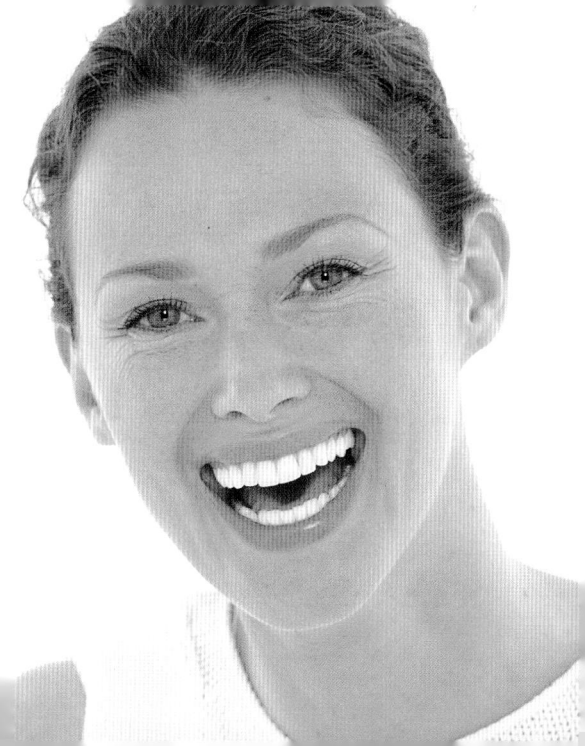

A smile can melt the hardest heart and wipe years off your face. Your mouth speaks volumes about you without making a single murmur, and as you speak, it frames every word you utter. Full and pouting – you are a sex-kitten, then thin and slightly turned down at the edges – you are the cat. Next to your eyes, lips are your most expressive facial feature. They can announce that you are happy or sad, annoyed or

introducing lips

alluring. They also have the power to disguise the way you feel, and to change your mood in an instant. The 'Look Good Feel Good' campaign for breast cancer awareness was among the first to discover how a woman's spirits could be lifted just by applying lipstick, even through illness and therapy. Lips are a most visible sensual part of our body – which is all the more reason why we should look after them.

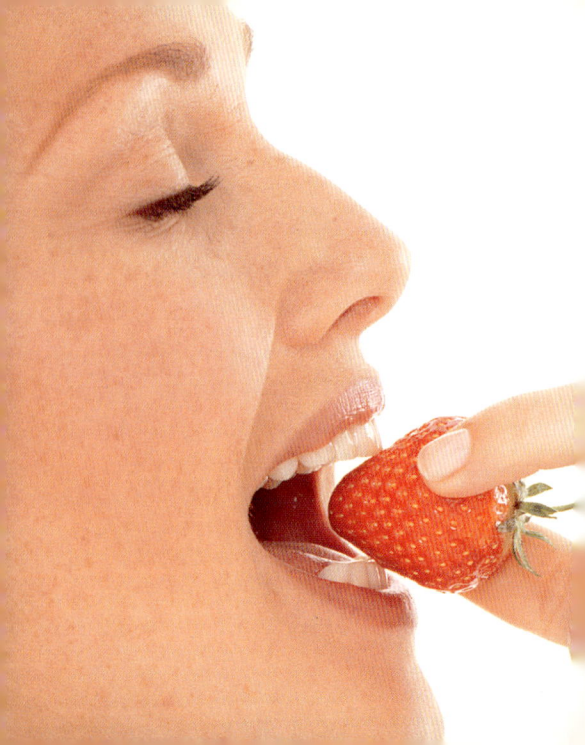

'...take, oh take, those lips away that so sweetly were foresworn.'

William Shakespeare

Lip colour is the finishing touch to your whole look, and the right colour can make all the difference to the way others perceive you. Think of Hollywood stars such as Mae West, Marlene Dietrich, Marilyn Monroe and Joan Crawford – they all made a sexy signature from their rich, red lips. Yet their starring roles were mostly in black-and-white movies. We did not need to see their actual lip colour, we just knew that it was rich and deep, and that it had to be red. In fact, female stars needed to lighten their hair and accentuate their lips if only to make themselves stand out more as the star on the black-and-white screen. This is still true today, as Sharon Stone made nude beige lips the 'in thing' with her part in the film *Basic Instinct*.

'... stand up straight and smile! It's the fastest way to take ten years off your looks.'

Dayle Haddon, model and author

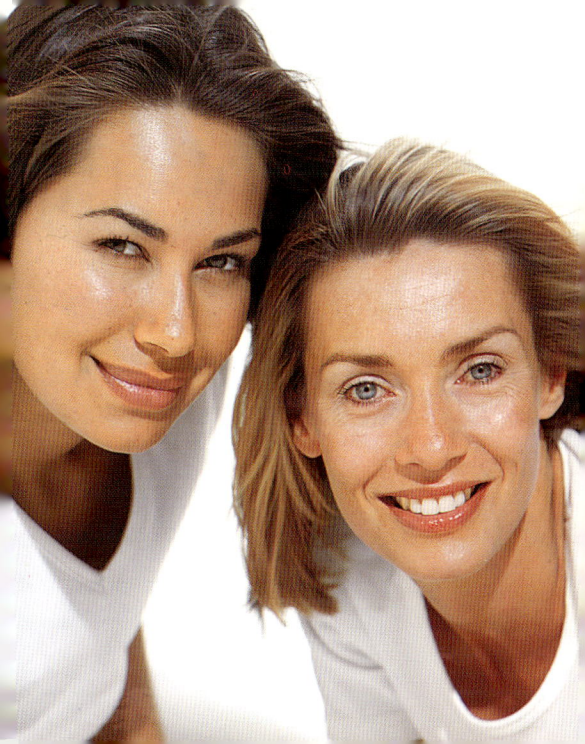

protect them, soften them, nourish them: the more attention you give your lips, the more attention you will receive in return

looking

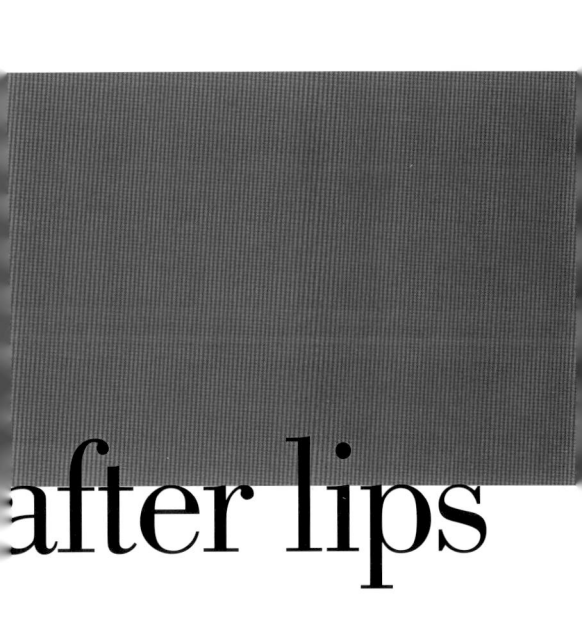

after lips

The skin on your lips is both thinner and finer than the skin on the rest of your face. It is even more vulnerable than the delicate skin around the eyes, lacking in several of the body's protective substances, including an affective lipidic barrier which helps to keep moisture in the skin, and keeps it soft and plump.

Lips need extra protection from the drying effects of the sun, wind, central heating and

giving lips extra help

air conditioning. They lose moisture regularly – licking your lips makes them even drier – and they contain no sebaceous glands to help keep them supple, which makes them more prone to dryness and chapping.

To keep lips soft, supple and younger looking for longer, regularly hydrate them with a lip balm or lip salve. These are made from fatty substances such as beeswax or carnuba

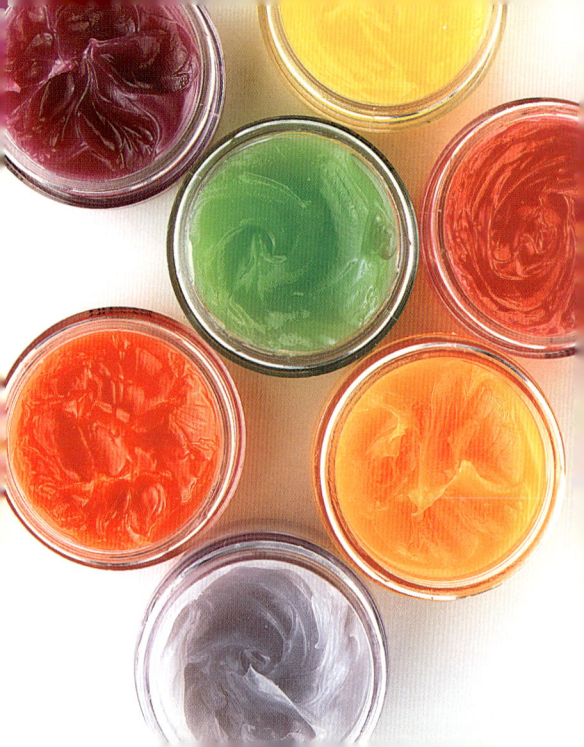

wax which seals the lips and acts as an invisible barrier to retain moisture. Make sure also that the surrounding skin is kept sufficiently moisturised to prevent lines from appearing around your mouth. Use a daily moisturiser that contains vitamins A, C and E and a sunscreen. This will help to protect skin from oxidative damage caused by free radicals that lead to premature ageing, particularly if you smoke.

You can find many lip balms and lipsticks now with a high Sun Protection Factor (SPF) to wear when you are outdoors – even in winter. This is considered by dermatologists as vital protection since the lips contain little or no melanin (the body's natural mechanism against sun), so are easily burned and damaged by the sun. Lips can burn easily and are a prime site for cold sores (encouraged by sun exposure).

Always protect them with a sun screen or lipstick, which acts as a sunscreen in itself due to its high powder content. Most of all be aware of the condition of your lips. Just like the rest of your skin, it's a barometer for the way you live your life. Try to increase your water intake (especially if your lips seem permanently dry), be less stressed (to avoid frown lines around the mouth), nourish and protect.

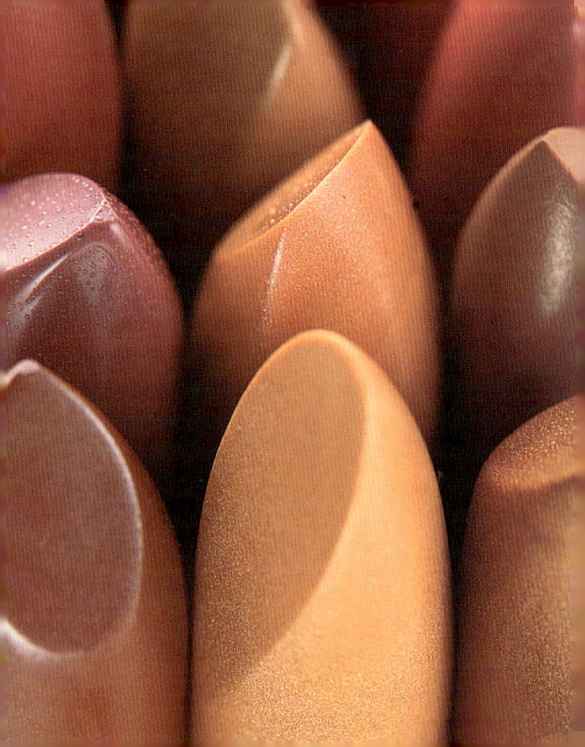

'when a woman goes out to buy a lipstick, it's as much fun as sex.'

BeneFit Cosmetics

As we get older, our lips lose some of their fat and so get thinner. The fragile skin around the lips becomes prone to fine lines, so as our body ages, our lips are one of the most vulnerable areas (next to eyes) in the continual fight against ageing.

There is a basic daily skin-care routine that you can practice, which if started when you are young, will keep your mouth and lips – and so your entire

lip-care plan

face – looking youthful for much longer.

Always protect your lips from sun exposure. UV light causes up to 90 per cent of skin ageing. Lipstick is one of the best sunscreens available. As a combination of waxes and powder particles, it blocks out as much sun as anything will, and the more intense the colour the better the protection. However, summer shades are often more sheer, so make sure that you take care to reapply regularly.

Look after your teeth. A winning smile might melt hearts, but if your teeth aren't in good condition, it can spoil the way you look and sap your confidence. The older we get the worse our teeth become, particularly if you drink tea, coffee or red wine and smoke cigarettes. If your teeth are already looking dull or yellow-brown in colour, try cutting

down on these. Brushing regularly after each meal for two minutes is essential, but a visit to the hygienist for professional cleaning is always a good investment and one which is becoming more commonplace in the UK.

A good diet is vital to maintain healthy skin and teeth. If you can't stop smoking completely, try to cut down and increase your intake of antioxidant vitamins A, C and E. Cigarette smoking releases skin-ageing free radicals into your body, breaking down the collagen and alastin that keep skin looking young and supple.

Finally, get a little laughter in to your life. It brings a light to your eyes and a smile to everyone's lips, especially yours. And let's face it, better to have lines later in life that turn up from a lifetime of laughter, than turn down from a life time of sorrow.

Look after your lips. Carry your usual skin care over to your lips as well. They need just as much care, if not more, and you can now buy moisturising masks and compresses specifically for lips.

Your lip's best friend is Vaseline petroleum jelly. If you suffer from chapped or scuffed lips apply Vaseline or lip balm regularly. Never tear at loose skin with your teeth, instead try our troubleshooting tips.

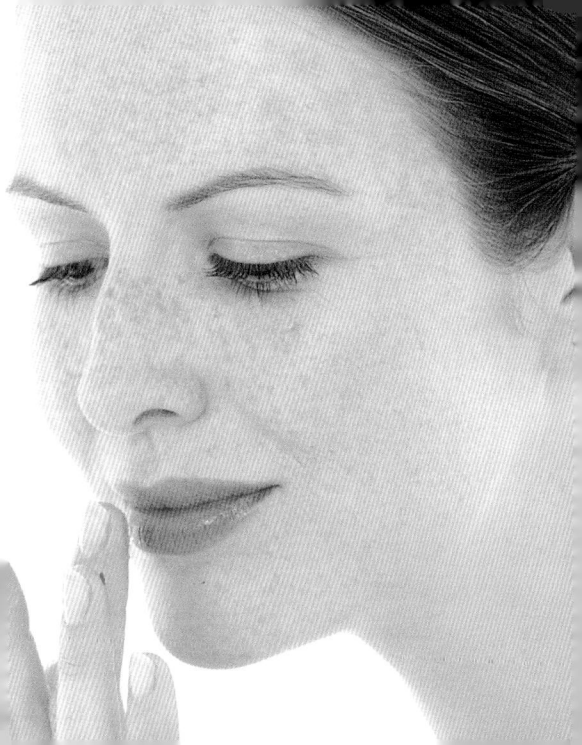

Lipstick is a woman's best friend – an item of make-up that even those of us who rarely use face powders or lotions may feel bare and uncomfortable without. Most lipsticks consist of a fatty base, to ensure that the product stays firm and spreads effectively. Colour is achieved using dyes or pigments. A good lipstick is soft enough to adhere to the lips smoothly and should stay put for some hours.

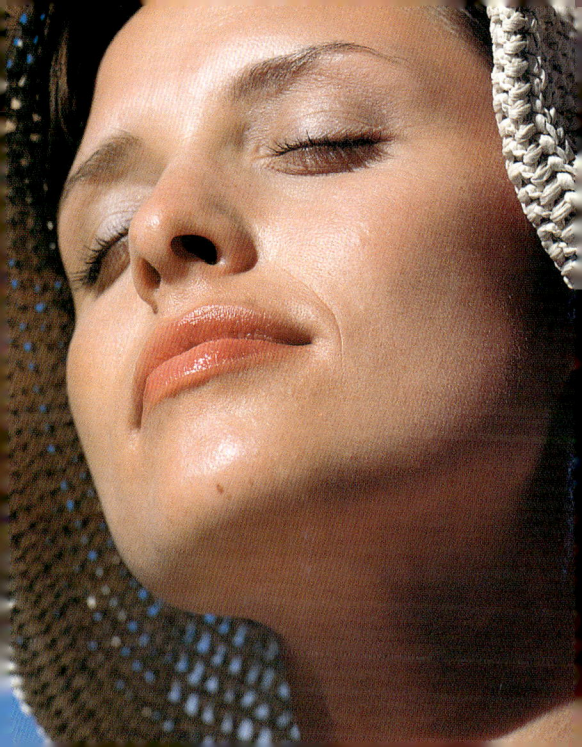

If your lips are dry or cracked – protect them with a lip balm containing a minimum SPF 15. Reapply as often as you remember throughout the day. Do not wait for them to get dry.

If you have fine lines around your mouth – make sure that you carry your usual moisturiser over your lips as part of your daily skin-care regime. Lip primers have a conditioning formula that also provides a no-bleed base for lipstick.

To accentuate your natural lip line and to hold colour in place throughout the day – use a lip pencil.

trouble-shooting lip care

- If you suffer from cold sores – use a sunscreen on your lips of no less than SPF 15. The sun stimulates the herpes virus, but with adequate protection you should find you suffer far less.
- For a DIY conditioning lip mask – give your lips a coat of vitamin E oil. Mix 5 ml of vitamin E oil with one drop of rose oil. It gives them an instant natural shine without colour and will condition and protect them too. Apply at night but never under lipstick, as oils make colour slide off in seconds.

'lipstick is the first thing a young girl reaches for when she plays with her mother's make-up.'

Bobbi Brown, make-up artist

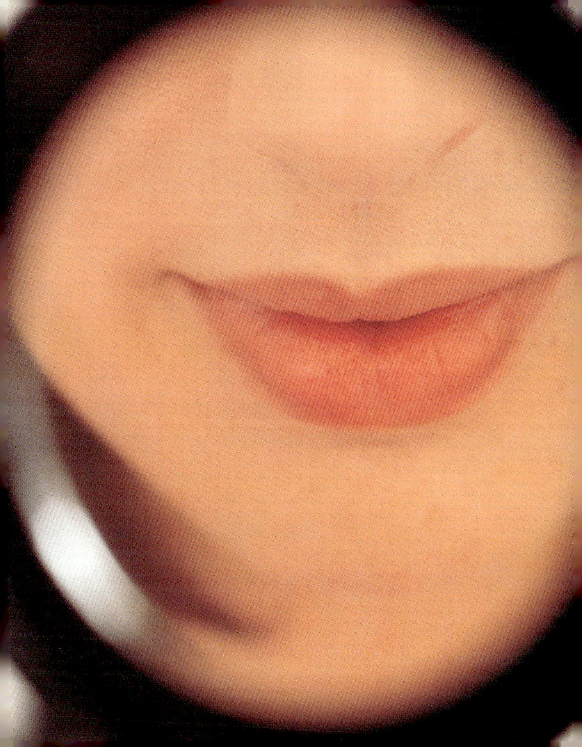

exercise is good for you,
so why not add in a fe
simple work-outs for
your lips and
jaw to your
fitness regime.

lip work

outs

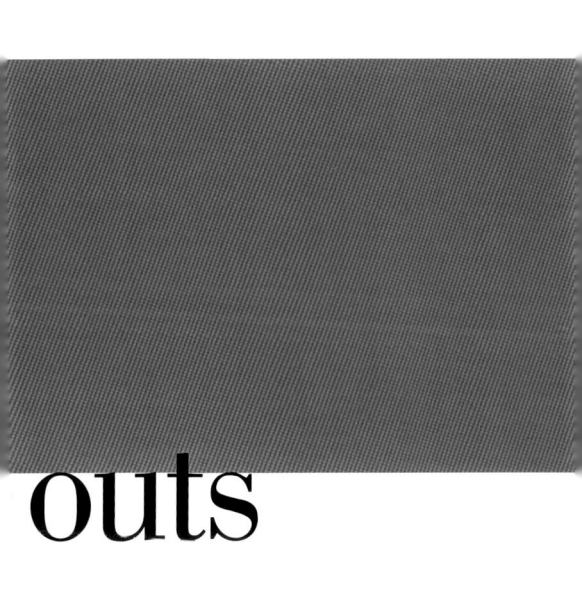

Talking, laughing and shouting on a daily basis should count as a daily work-out in itself, yet some specific facial work-out routines are said to exercise certain muscle groups which help to keep your face firm and youthful looking. If nothing else, a facial work-out is a great way to relieve tension in areas such as the jaw.

To get the most out of these exercises, sit comfortably in a chair, face a mirror, and

focus on your lips

completely relax. To make each exercise fully effective, you need to carry out each movement as slowly as possible and as if you are working against resistance. Try these exercises first thing in the morning to help you feel energised and fully awake. Another bonus is that over time these movements may help to avoid negative expression lines such as pursed lips and a downturned mouth.

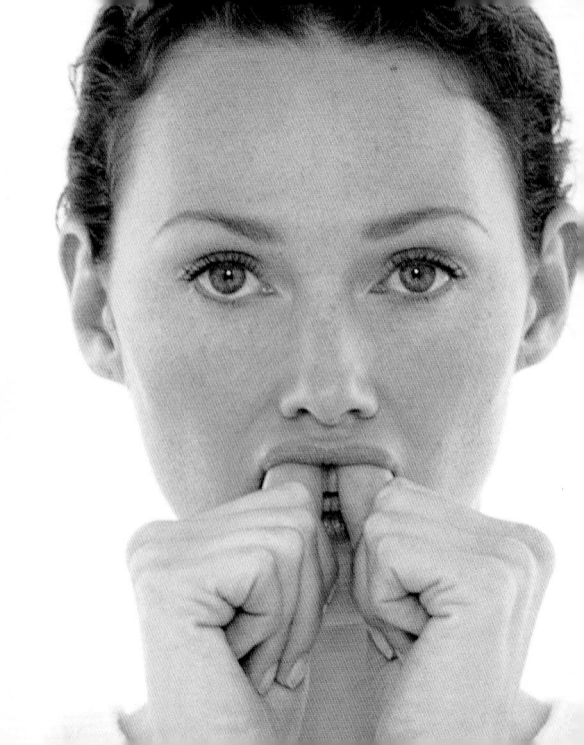

Lip-line eraser – with elbows on a table, look straight ahead and place both thumbs under your top lip with the nails resting against your upper teeth and gum. In one slow movement, gently move your upper lip muscles toward your thumbs, hold for a count of five, then slowly release. Repeat 15 times.

Lower lip and chin exercise – with your mouth in an 'O' shape, place the tips of your thumb and index finger between your top and bottom lip. The pads of your fingers should be facing each other and be about 2cm (¾in) apart. Then for 15–30 seconds try to make your thumb and index finger touch using your lips only, but keep them resisting the pressure.

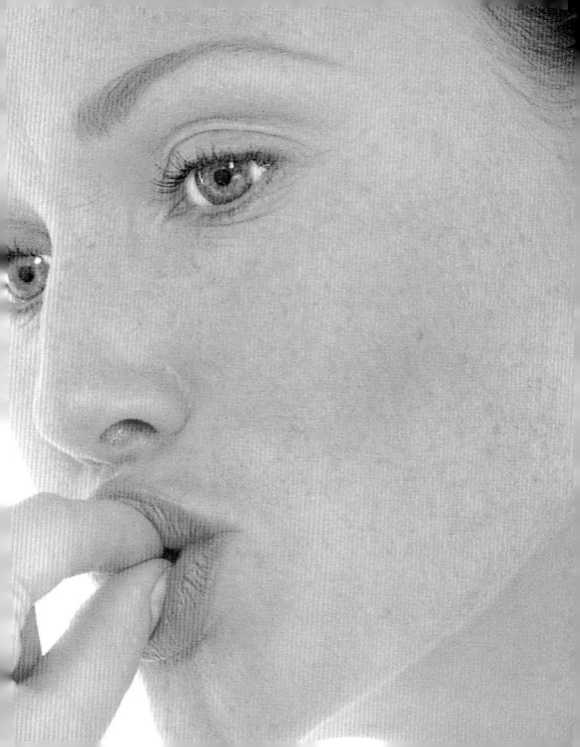

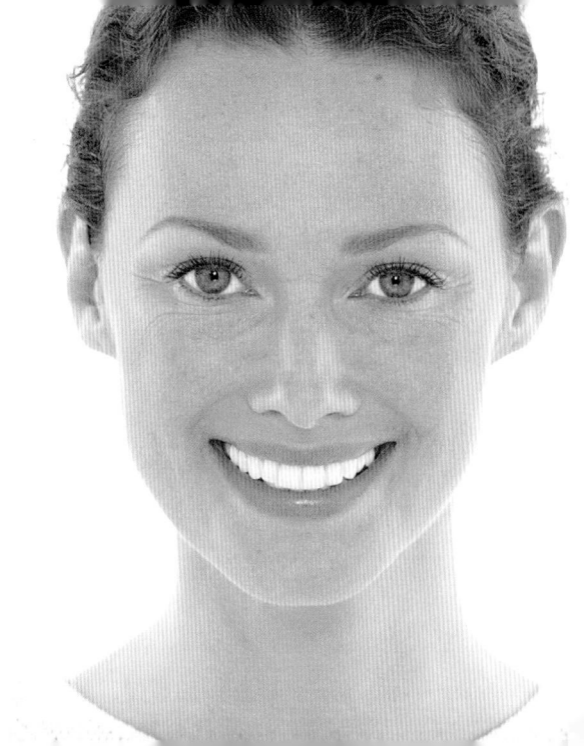

Smile aerobics – keeping your mouth slightly open, smile repeatedly every second, repeat 20–30 times. This will help to prevent the sides of your mouth from turning down by strengthening your jaw muscles.

Say your vowels – A, E, I, O, U. Do this 15–20 times as a great pick-me-up when you are feeling tired. Say them very slowly and exaggerate each vowel as you say it.

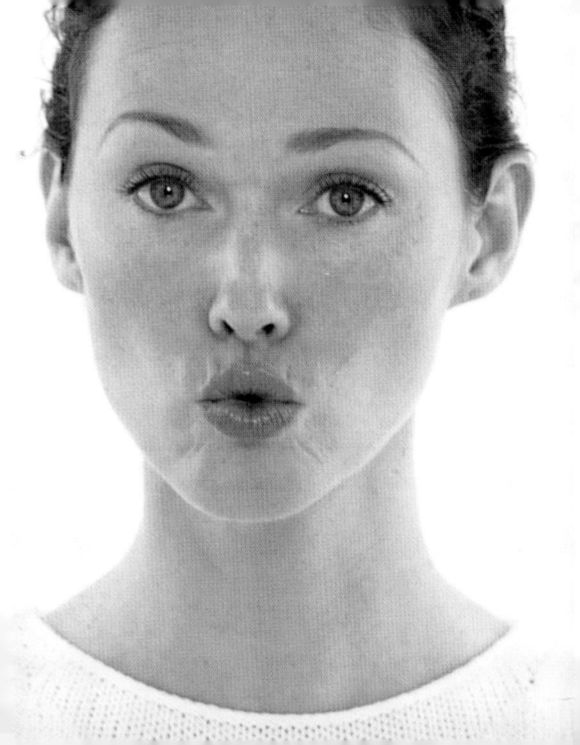

whether sheer and glossy or rich and well-defined, good-looking lips that are well cared for give you the image of being well groomed.

making

p lips

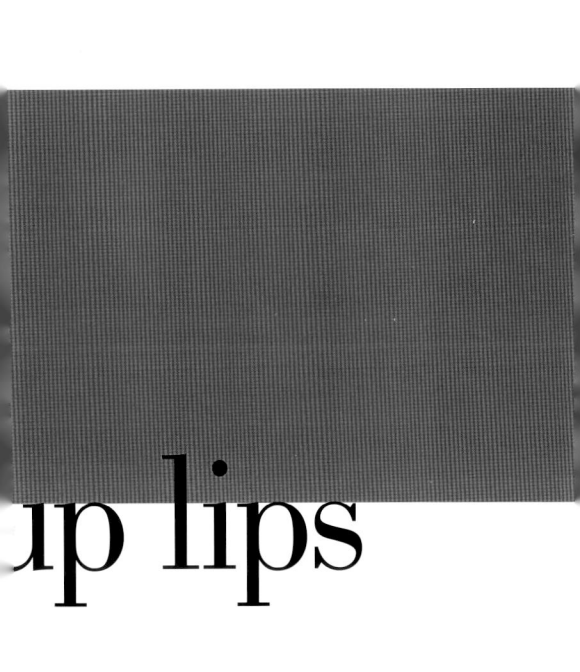

Well looked-after lips are far more appealing than those with a slap-dash slick of colour that's uneven and smudged. It does not have to take much thought, just a bit of practice until it becomes second nature. How well your lipstick goes on and remains put has a lot to do with the way you prime your lips before applying your lip colour. Dry, dehydrated lips invariably soak up emollients and leave behind an uneven

priming your lips

stain. Lips that are too moist will lose even the longest-lasting formula in seconds because the lip colour will have no base on which to cling.

A lip primer will condition lips while giving colour a base upon which to set. It's an extra step in your regime, but might be worth the effort if you find your lipstick disappears fast.

To ensure the best application, prepare your lips first with a smear of moisturising lip balm.

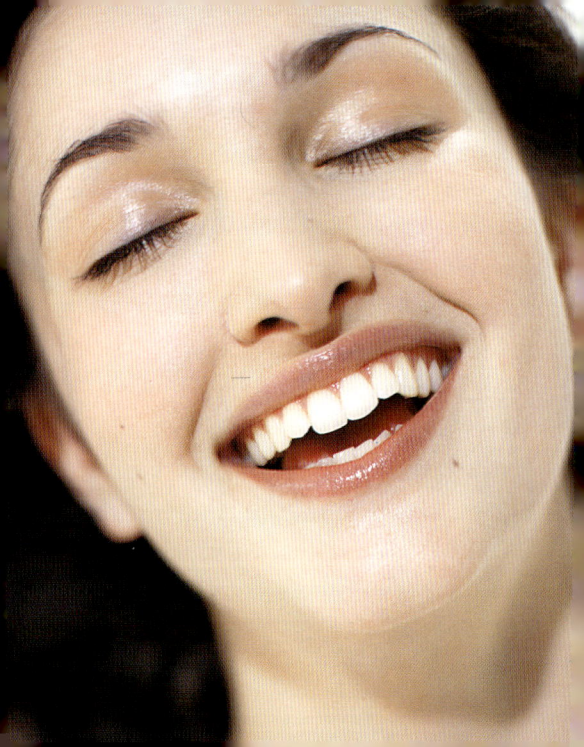

Apply over your lips at the beginning of your make-up, and leave to absorb while you do the rest of your face. After finishing the rest of the face, blot off any excess balm with a tissue. Lips will look smooth – but not so slick that colour disappears in seconds.

Tip: for a steady hand when applying lipstick rest your elbow on a table, particularly when doing the initial outline.

Outline your lips to give them the stronger definition they may need. Fill in an uneven outline with a good lip pencil; its firm consistency will prevent lipstick from bleeding into any surrounding fine lines or wrinkles around your mouth. Start by tracing the pencil along the actual lip-line itself. Avoid trying to draw outside your natural lip line, or you will end up with a very unattractive rim around your

defining your lips

mouth once the lip colour begins to fade.

Make-up artists recommend drawing either inside your natural lip-line, to make lips look thinner, or outside it, to make them look fuller. Then, in order to make a pencilled mouth look less crisp, run a dry brush around the edge to soften the line.

For a longer lasting finish, you can colour in the entire lip area with pencil instead of using lipstick. Use the side of the pencil to fill in, then soften with a coat of lip balm to prevent your lips from drying out. A chubby lip pencil will not create a good lip contour. It will have a creamy formulation and smudge easily. Keep one for emergency colour only.

Tip: in warm climates, submerge lip pencils (with caps on) in ice water to keep tips firm.

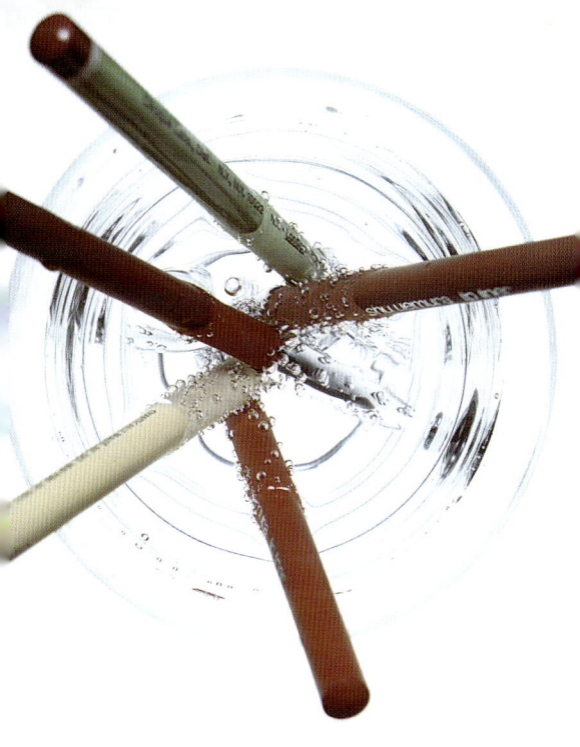

One minute it's neutrals, the next it's reds. Then, just as we get into glossy, along comes matte again.

Choosing the lip colour to suit your complexion is not easy. Think about the kind of look you want to create – whether to wear a dark dramatic mouth, a pretty pastel-pink mouth or a natural 'barely-there-at-all' mouth.

How do you choose? Hold a lip colour up to your face and if its tone flatters your hair and skin colour, consider it.

choosing a lip colour

Deep, rich colours warm the complexion, while pale colours drain it. Therefore, if you choose a colour somewhere between the two for a daytime shade, your job of selection will be made much easier.

Pink-brown shades that closely match your actual lip colour suit almost everyone and give the most natural look.

Brown and toffee tones are flattering too, offering subtle definition without being garish.

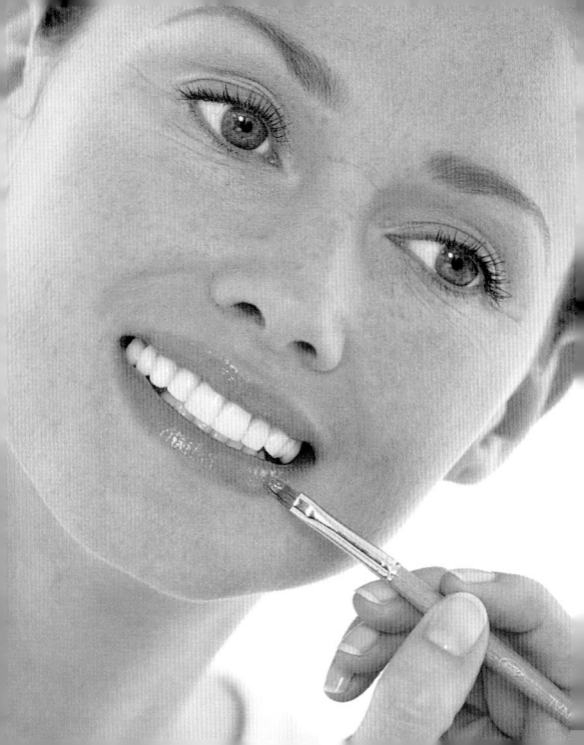

■ Red lipstick needs precise application and a certain amount of confidence to carry it off. Remember that red lipstick can appear harsh against fair skin.
■ Blue-toned reds and pinks can look harsh on fair or older skins. If in doubt, go for golden, yellow-toned colours that illuminate the skin.

Tip: test out a new colour on the pad of your fingertip, as skin colour here is similar to the colour of your lips.

There are no hard and fast rules to choosing a new lip colour except that you should always feel comfortable in your chosen colour. Remember also that you are wearing the lip colour, it should not overpower your natural looks. Here are some colour pointers for natural and coloured hair to go with your skin type.

Blond hair

fair skin: daytime – light brown; evening – plum
olive skin: daytime – raisin; evening – red
dark skin: daytime – plum; evening – red

lip-colour chart

Red hair

fair skin: daytime – natural; evening – spice

olive skin: daytime – russet; evening – plum

dark skin: daytime – brown; evening – wine

Brown-black hair

fair skin: daytime – plum; evening – wine-red

olive skin: daytime – berry; evening – browny red

dark skin: daytime – damson; evening – blackberry

Grey hair

fair skin: daytime – rose-pink; evening – fuchsia

olive skin: daytime – browny red; evening – red

dark skin: daytime – berry; evening – magenta

Would you rather have luscious, succulent lips with a sexy, glossy sheen, or a well-defined matte mouth that stays in place all day?

The colour of your lipstick is season-led so that in summer your lipstick, like everything else, is sheer and shimmery to reflect not just the sunlight but also the overall mood of optimism. Come winter, however, you can guarantee that fashion colours become deeper, richer,

lip effects and textures

matte and more defined, to go with heavier fabrics and darker hues.

Think about what you like and what you want from your lipstick. If you like glossy lip colour but you are over 50, place the gloss only in the centre of the bottom lip where it will look more sophisticated and flattering than all-over colour. If you have thin lips enhance them with a coloured lip balm or shimmer shade.

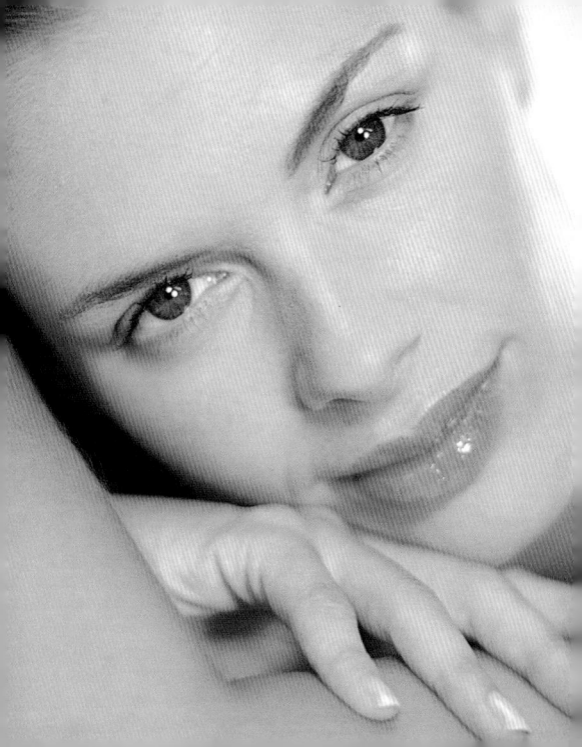

Gloss gives lips a soft and youthful look and keeps lips feeling smoother than a lipstick does. Use either a clear gloss or Vaseline and apply over the top of your lip-colour. Wear gloss to highlight your lips or to enhance their natural colour. Dab it on the centre of the top and bottom lips and press lips together – this way, you will get the illusion of all-over gloss without the slip factor.

Matte lipstick contains a high percentage of powder and although this is what makes it long-lasting you might find you want something a little less flat. There is a new generation of longer lasting lip-colours that use polymers and silicones to remove the dryness.

Tip: try mixing matte lipstick with a little lip balm. It will not last as long, but your lips will feel more comfortable.

Cream lipstick gives the sensuous appeal of a full, youthful mouth. The smooth texture of cream lipstick allows you to wear darker shades that appear softer, prettier and more flattering. The best way to apply creamy formulas is to blot the first layer with a tissue, then reapply with a lip brush. In this way, the first coat stains your lips a little, which then helps the second coat to stay in place better.

You can apply lip colour straight from the bullet, with a lip-wand and with your fingertips, but none of these gives you the control and accuracy of a lip brush.

No professional make-up artist would be without a lip brush – it allows colour to be spread evenly over the lips, enables colour to stay on longer and, because you don't overload your lips with colour, you inevitably use less lipstick.

brush talk

Brushes give a softer look to lip liner because they enable you to blend away any harsh obvious edges.

Make sure you purchase a retractable lip brush – one that has its own case so it's easy to carry around and stays clean. Otherwise look for a slim flat brush with flexible bristles that should be about 8mm (⅓in) long – neither too short or too long to control, nor too short to be hard and inflexible.

Try these top lipstick tricks known to the professionals for great effects.

Caught without your lipstick? Do not go bare, do as the make-up artists do, and use anything you have to hand. Rub on a little rosy blusher or some toffee-coloured shadow then seal with lip balm.

Only ever use a lip liner that is three or four shades darker than the natural colour of your lips.

To prevent a harsh lip line, try applying lip liner after your lipstick. This way the pencil will blend more easily and will not stand out and look obvious.

lipstick tricks

- Buy a selection of about five lipsticks and achieve hundreds of colours. If you have one true pink, one deep-brown, one pillar-box red, a clear orange and a pearly, translucent one, you can create any lipstick colour you desire.
- If you find the price of lipsticks too hard to bear and cannot face throwing out your old lipstick stubs get a small tin or old eye-shadow compact and scoop out the remaining lip colour. Then, simply apply with your fingertips for a soft undefined mouth or with a lip brush for more precision.

If your natural lip line is uneven – you will find a lip pencil indispensable. Choose a shade that matches the colour of your lips and carefully draw around the line of your mouth. Do not leave an obvious line, but gently blend it into your lips. Then apply any colour you like, even just a clear lip gloss.

If you get lipstick on your teeth, do what models do – place your index finger in your mouth, close your lips around it, and pull your finger out. Any lipstick that might have ended up on your teeth, comes off on your finger.

trouble-shooting lipstick

- If you have drawn a wobbly outline – blot your lips with a tissue and use a cotton bud to clean up the lip contour. Next, apply a little of your usual concealer over the entire lip line and pat and blend. Then apply a light dusting of face powder and, with a steady hand, redo your lip line.
- If you suffer from flaky lips – do the well-known tooth-brush trick. Rub Vaseline all over your lips and gently buff away at the flakes with an old, clean toothbrush. It's the oldest trick in the book, but nothing has surpassed it yet.

If you have lines around your mouth and your lipstick bleeds and feathers – prepare the skin around the mouth first with a moisturiser to smooth out the lines. Then use a lip pencil to define the outline of your lips and give the lipstick something else on which to adhere. Remember to powder your lips well before and after applying colour.

- If you are in a rush – apply a neutral pink-brown lip colour rather than red or some other deep-coloured lipsticks that require more lengthy and precise application.
- If your mouth is small – enhance your lips by applying a light-reflective concealer all over the lip contour so the real lip line is less defined. Leave your own lip alone but try extending the lines of your upper lip out at the corners.

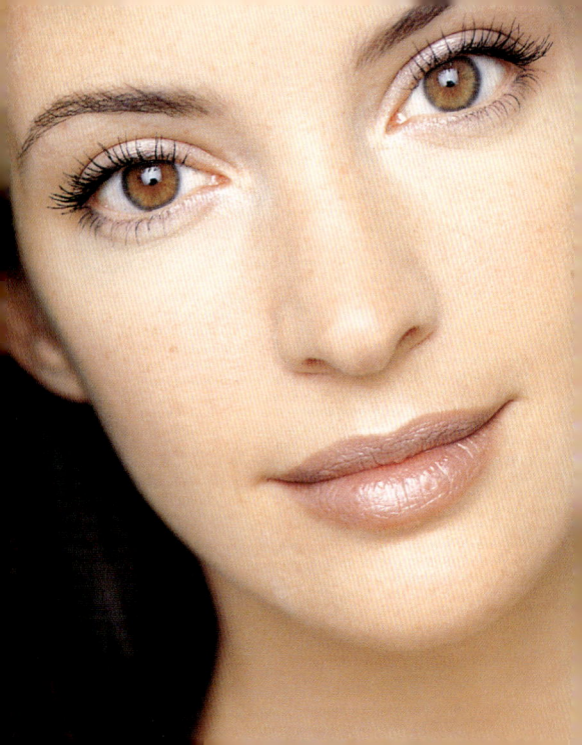

'...lipstick can make a woman look sexier, sweeter, bolder ... more glamorous ...'

Bobbi Brown, make-up artist

here are a few new ways
to give your lips
a new look,
and play with their
natural shape to
emphasise them.

lip looks

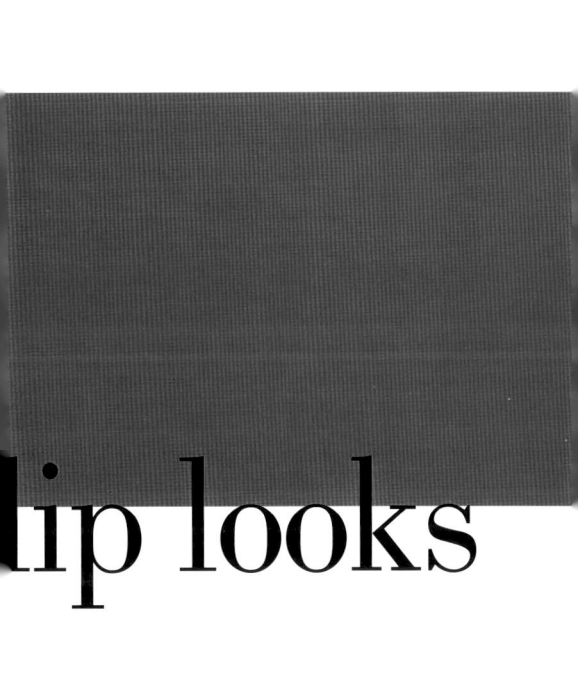

The majority of women tend to find one favourite lip colour and stick with it for years, applying it straight from the bullet. It's safe, easy and understandable, but that does not make it right. Lipstick does much, much more.

Create your ideal lip shape by using lip colour to subtly change the shape of your mouth and create illusions, from a pert little Cupid's bow to a full, strong outline.

creating your lip shape

Corrections are most effective if a subdued colour is used so that the new lip line looks soft and natural. Red is one of the worst shades to use when creating a new lip shape because it's bright and draws attention to the mouth, and therefore the false lip shape. Likewise, very glossy formulations are not especially effective either, as they reflect the light and alter the illusion you are trying to create. The best tones are matte, medium shades that closely resemble the natural colour and texture of your lips when left bare.

When you are changing the natural shape of your mouth, do not try to alter the entire lip line – the fakery will just become more obvious as the colour fades away. You can block out your natural lip shape by using a foundation stick or concealer to match the surrounding skin tone. Then practice redesigning your lips with lip pencil (again, in a tone that matches your natural lip colour), drawing in the shape you want, going inside or outside the natural line. Never overdo it, minor adjustments done thoughtfully and carefully are far more convincing.

Most of us would like to have a fuller mouth, especially as we get older and our lips get thinner. Avoid creating a lip line where you would like it to be, rather than where it should be – you will only end up looking like a clown. The best way to enhance the shape of your lips is to apply a layer of light-reflective concealer all over the lip area and onto the skin. It will magically illuminate the whole area and make your lips

full lips

appear fuller. Next, draw your lip line with a firm pencil just a fraction beyond the natural edge of your lips, then soften the edge of the line with your finger tip or with a dry lip brush. Finally, fill the whole area in with a medium matte shade of lipstick (too dark a shade will only make your lips appear smaller) and add a dab of gloss to the centre of the bottom lip to make it appear bigger and more rounded.

Finishing tip: when the mouth is soft in a medium shade of lipstick, everything else should balance out, so give definition to eyes with liner and mascara and use plenty of blusher.

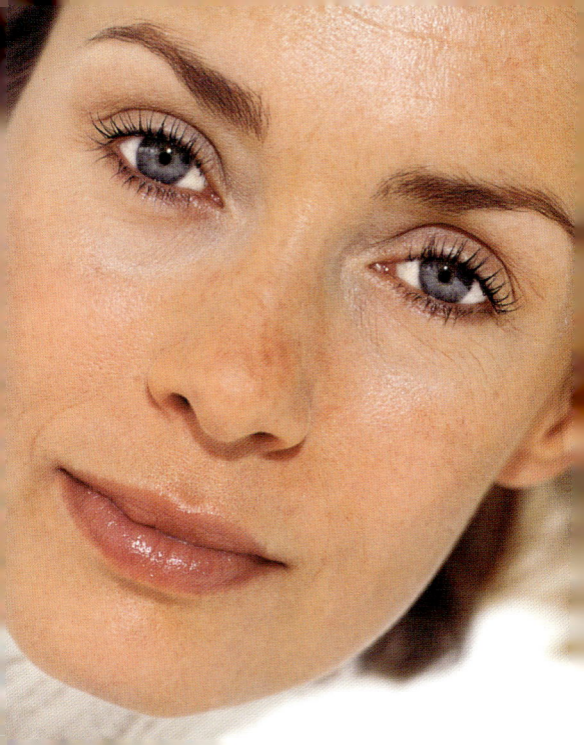

To make lips look more full and rounded, prime lips with foundation and powder. Then take a neutral colour lip pencil and draw a shape slightly outside the natural lip line, along the top and bottom but without emphasising the corners. Next, take a lighter shade of lipstick and apply it to the middle of both the top and bottom lips. Now you have defined the outline of your lips, blend the two together by filling in with the

sexy pout

pencil or a slightly darker lip colour, keeping the colour lighter in the centre of the lips to give the illusion of a fuller mouth. Then you can put lip gloss on top, but again only on the centre section. Try a shimmering silver lip gloss that has more impact for evening. This way you will achieve a neutral finish that looks sexy and natural, and will not get a harsh line around the lips, from the lip liner.

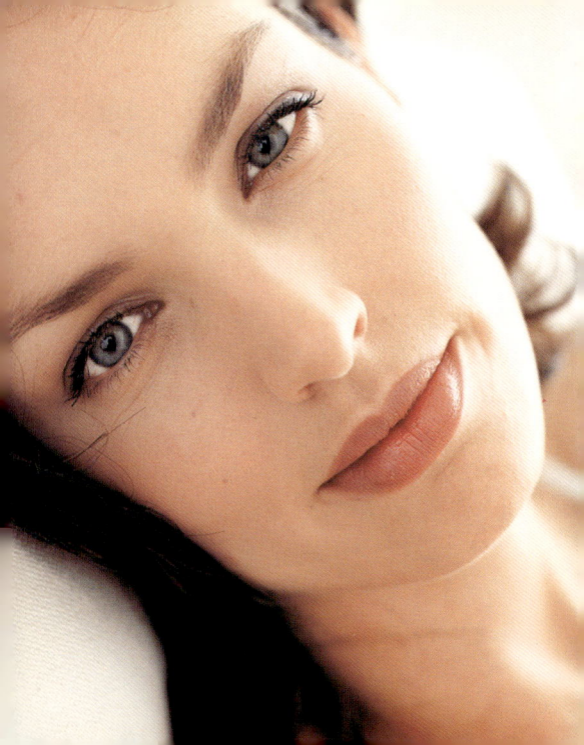

Finishing tip: when you want your lips to look full, rounded and attract all the attention, go for a minimum amount of eye make-up – say, only mascara. Avoid wearing any shimmer highlighter around the eyes, it will only detract from lips you've so carefully created.

Begin by priming your lips with a foundation stick or concealer so that your natural lip line is softened. Then powder your lips; to create a Cupid's bow you need the colour to stay in place as long as possible. For the perfect lip shape, start by drawing a reference point in the middle of the 'M' of your upper lip, then one on each point and finally one in the middle of the lower lip line. Join the three points of the

cupid's bow

'M'. Starting from the corners and with an open smile, trace the lip outline to join the points in the middle. Lightly blend it towards the inside of the lips with a lip brush to soften the effect. Your choice of lip colour will no doubt be quite bold, and in this instance, choose a lip liner to match, so that as it starts to wear off, it is easy to fill in quickly without having to redraw the shape. Check how it looks in a mirror throughout

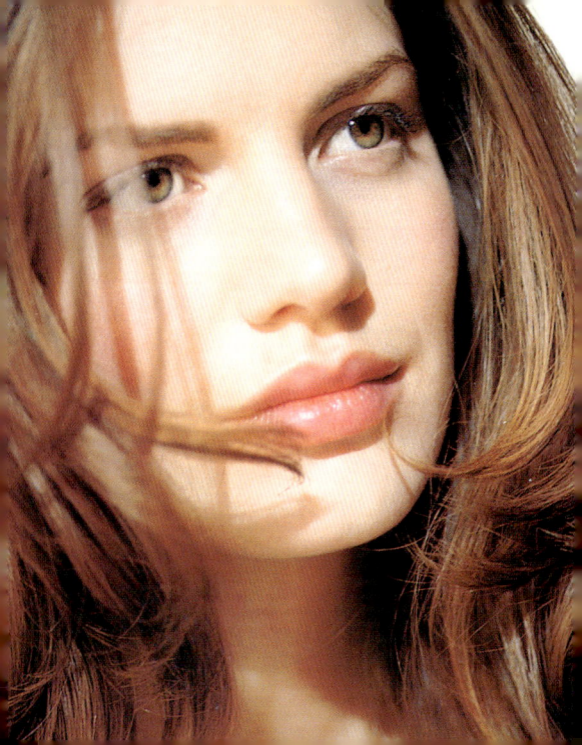

the day, you need to replenish this look often for it to look really good.

Finishing tip: the overall effect when drawing in the Cupid's bow is very dramatic. Keep the eyes simple so that they neither detract from the lips, nor conflict in drama.

Go for gloss and pale colours. Any rule about women of a certain age not wearing gloss has been put to bed by make-up artists who believe that anything goes, so long as it's applied in the right way. Be sparing with the gloss and the effect will be much prettier. Prime your lips as usual, then apply lip-liner pencil in a neutral tone all over your lips first. Carry the colour over your lips as a bolder base, then

young soft lips

soften the contour edge with a clean lip brush to soften the line. Take a sheer, pink-tinted lip gloss and apply to the middle of the bottom lip only, then press lips together. Do not take the shine right up to the lip line or the look will appear over done.

Make-up artists live by this rule: when you are going for gloss, keep everything else subtle. When you've created eye catching glossy lips, keep your eye make-up minimal and matte, and your cheeks soft and rosy. That way you'll stay looking younger and fresh.

Finishing tip: as an option for the evening, try applying a shimmer stick on upper cheekbones and along the jawbone, use the Cupid's bow for your lips. This gives back the bloom to the skin – your natural sheen.

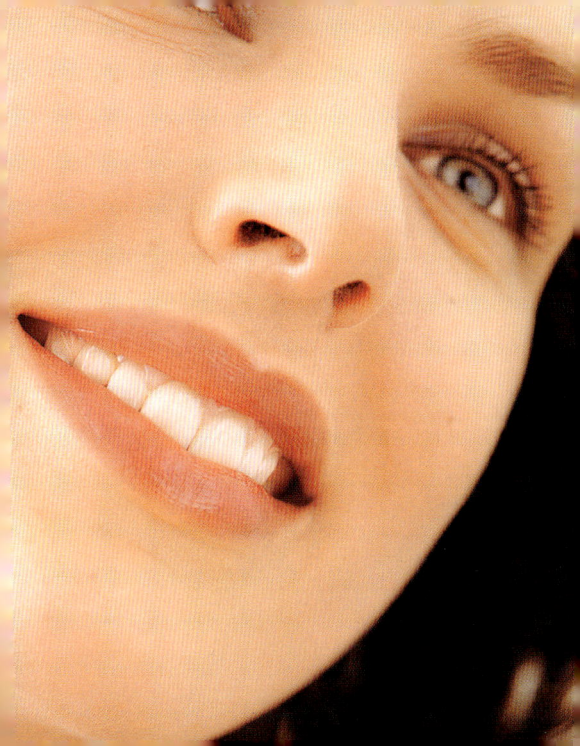

The trick is in covering up parts of the lips that appear too big. To make a mouth appear smaller, you need to blend foundation over the natural edge and down onto the lips and apply powder so it sets in place. Then pencil a false line just a fraction inside the true shape of your mouth and fill it in with a deep-toned lip colour such as plum or berry. Avoid very pale or very bright tones as these will draw more

slimming down full lips

attention to your lips. Stick to matte colours too, as shimmery textures will make the lips appear bigger. Finally blot the lips with a tissue to reduce the impact of the colour still further and make your new mouth appear more natural.

Remember, if you are trying to detract from your lips, you should always emphasise your eyes instead. Wear an extra coat of mascara and place a shimmery highlighter on the brows so they catch the light, and everyone else's eyes, first.

Finishing tip: if you are trying to detract from your lips, make your eyes the focal point. Use a highlighter on the brows so they catch the light, invest in sparkling eye drops, get your brows shaped or your lashes curled – whatever it takes to make your eyes catch the eye of others first.

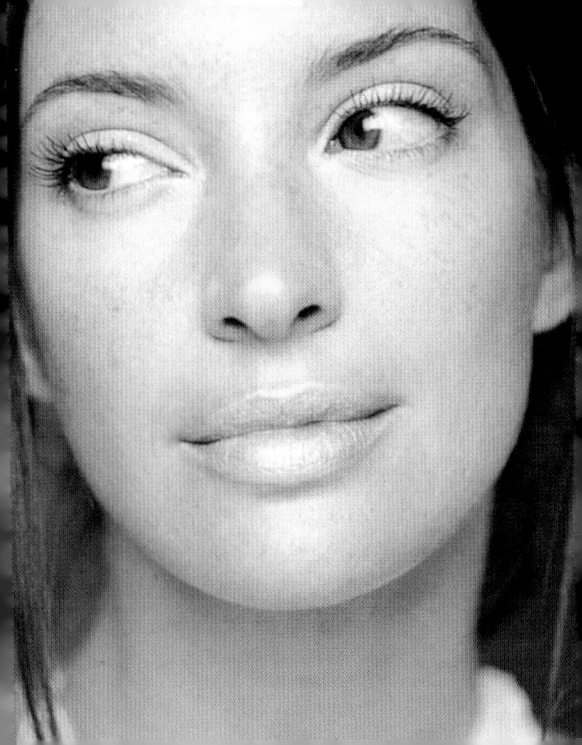

Bold, strong lip colour instantly gives a smart elegant and dressy look. Most women tend to choose a classic red for evening, but variations such as burgundy, damson and brown-red look equally stunning. A creamy formulation gives just the right amount of shimmer without looking glossy. Apply foundation and powder over your mouth as you would the rest of your face, to give lipstick a cleaner surface and

glamorous lips

better hold. When applying a strong colour always use a lip pencil as it helps to keep the edges neat and prevents the colour from feathering. Draw a soft outline in a matching pencil and keep as close to your natural lip line as possible. Paint on one layer, using a lipbrush, blot with a tissue, then reapply and blot again. This way the colour acts more like a stain, and stays on your lips for longer.

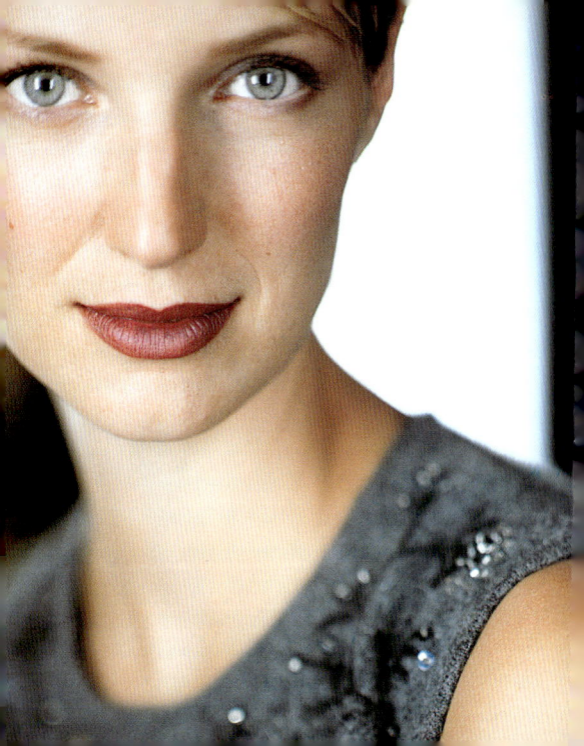

Finishing tip: balance a dark, sophisticated mouth with subtle but defined eye make-up. Light eye-shadow, dark lashes and groomed brows ensure an elegant, glamorous make-up that looks fresh and modern too.

First published in 2000 by
HarperCollins*Illustrated*
An imprint of HarperCollins*Publishers*
77–85 Fulham Palace Road
London W6 8JB

The HarperCollins website address is: www.**fire**and**water**.com

Published in association with The National Magazine Company Limited.
Good Housekeeping is a registered trademark of The National Magazine Company
Limited and the Hearst Corporation.

The Good Housekeeping website address is www.goodhousekeeping.co.uk

Copyright © 2000 HarperCollins*Illustrated*

All photographs are the copyright of the National Magazine Company Limited
with the following exceptions: Maureen Barrymore (pp 5, 9, 27, 31, 42, 45, 46, 49
and 62) and Derek Lomas (cover photograph, pp. 18, 22 and 59). Special thanks to
Liz Brown and Jane Bradley.

All rights reserved. No part of this publication may be reproduced, stored in
a retrieval system or transmitted, in any form or by any means, electronic,
mechanical photocopying, recording or otherwise, without the prior written
permission of the publisher.

British Library Cataloguing-in-Publication Data
A catalogue record for this book is available from the British Library.
ISBN 0-00-710461-8

Colour reproduction by Colourscan, Singapore
Printed and bound in China by Imago